Definitely Yours!
Keith 12/3/99

Deaf Proverbs

A Proverbial Professor's Points to Ponder

By Ken Glickman

Published by ***DEAFinitely Yours Studio***
9201 Long Branch Parkway, Silver Spring, Maryland 20901
http://www.deafology.com

Deaf Proverbs
First Edition

Also by Ken Glickman

DEAFinitions for SIGNLETS, the first volume
> Library of Congress Catalog Card Number 86-72758
> ISBN 0-9617583-0-9

***More DEAFinitions!*, the second volume**
> Library of Congress Catalog Card Number 89-50119
> ISBN 0-9617583-1-7

***DEAFinitions Galore!*, the third volume**
> Library of Congress Catalog Card Number 99-070651
> ISBN 0-9617583-3-3

DEAFinitions, poster
> Copyright 1986 by *DEAFinitely Yours Studio*

Play It by the Ear, poster
> Copyright 1989 by *DEAFinitely Yours Studio*

Copyright © 1999 by *DEAFinitely Yours Studio*
Library of Congress Catalog Card Number 99-070652
ISBN 0-9617583-2-5 Softcover
ISBN 0-9617583-4-1 Hardcover

ATTENTION — Organizations and Educational Institutions

Quantity discounts on bulk purchases of this book for fundraising and educational purposes are available. For information, please contact *DEAFinitely Yours Studio*, 9201 Long Branch Parkway, Silver Spring, Maryland 20901-3642 USA or email a note to Ken at ProfGlick@deafology.com (website: http://www.deafology.com).

All rights reserved. No part of this publication may be reproduced in any form
or by any means without prior permission in writing from the publisher.
- Proudly printed in the United States of America -

*Dedicated
to
all the inhabitants of the Deaf World
and those of you who are willing
to think Deaf.*

Acknowledgments with Thanks

My parents, **Lillian and Charles** - for their love and for instilling in me many tidbits of wisdom over the years.

My brother and sister, **Tom and Karen** - for being part of my two worlds.

Debbie Garcia - for her great, tender patience while I was deeply engrossed in writing this book.

Erin Sanborn - for her most wonderful book design work; one of the best birthday gifts for which any author could wish.

Gunam Emmanuel, Anita Farb, Karen Kimmel, Jennifer Nelson and Mary Truland - for their most constructive comments while proofreading this book.

April & Paul Rosenfeld, Claude Stout and Frank Tempesta - for their unfaltering encouragement and support.

Tony Toledo - for his love of books, one of which caught my eye and prompted me to write this one.

Wolfgang Mieder - for his numerous scholarly works on proverbs that provided me a lot of inspiration.

Kevin McLeod and Michele Westfall Listisard - for being such great "pounding" boards and for all their enthusiastic "Bingo!" comments that kept me going.

And my dog, **Star** - for our many leisurely walks, during which I let my mind wander.

Thank you, and enjoy the book!

Ken Glickman
Silver Spring, Maryland
May 15, 1999

Deaf Proverbs

The Deafie
who discovers the Deafie world
discovers himself.

Teach your child how to sign — for there is no finer gift than a hand-me-down.

A shoulder tap begets either a smile or a puzzled look.

Signs never fall on deaf ears.

Put your hands into motion once your brain is in gear.

Borrowing one's eyes draws interest.

What is signed cannot be unsigned.

Put a cap on one's abilities,
you get capabilities.

She may be deaf as a door knob, but that's only a small part of the whole thing.

Sign or face the music.

The hearly bird catches the word.

Empty-handedness betrays no one.

Small potatoes have big eyes.

A designer is
a signer sans signs.

One who listens with eyes is not so deaf.

Talk might be cheap,
but sign is steep.

One less sense,
each sense the greater.

Talking with one's back
to a bright window blinds —
otherwise, it illuminates.

Put your money where your hand is.

Calling one disabled
is half-empty;
Calling one capabled
is half-full.

Applause and upplause
sound the same
and are appreciated alike.

The school of hard knocks is a happy one.

Give your Hearie children
wings so they can fly
in both worlds.

White light
is better received than
any of its rainbow colors.

Sign little
and watch much.

Disarm a Deafie,
and you get a designer.

Sound the alarm,
you clear some;
Pound the floor,
you clear all.

A sign to the wise says it all.

Let noise be silvery,
for silence is golden.

Love is deaf.

Clip one's wings,
he cannot fly.

A sign a day keeps the teacher away.

To reach out to a friend, touch.

The right side is always
the bright side.

A road with signs is better traveled than one without.

Sleeping in pure silence recharges like none other.

Loose lips sink signs.

Never talk with your hands full.

When the deaf lead the deaf,
both walk side-by-side.

Pound to sound Deafies.

Light attracts,
dark repels.

Marry a Deafie, snore;
Marry a Hearie, tiptoe.

A sign in the hand is worth two in the book.

Stars unheard

are easy to see.

The sign is mightier than the word.

When there are too many eyes, keep your hands shut.

Keep your signs soft and sweet — in case you have to eat them.

Total communication
is greater than
the sum of ten supple fingers
and one big mouth.

Re-sign or resign.

Stand under light and you will understand.

Deafness is invisible
until you open your hands.

A sound sleep
is a soundless sleep.

Light travels faster and farther than sound.

Windows have eyes.

Street talk and street signs are not the same.

Expect lip service from glib terps.

A guessture
is a happy medium between
a real sign and a forgotten one.

When arguing with a Deafie, face it or it gets harder.

Deaf-impaired
is a Hearie who calls
Deafies hearing-impaired.

Handicap is for golfers only.

Signing never strikes twice in the same place.

Flowers belong to topsoil, not tabletops.

Money talks,
so teach it signs.

When money signs, the world keeps silent.

It is easier
to turn out the lights than
to stop gossip.

A wise head keeps one's hands still.

A sign learned one at a time is a good sign.

Silence sprinkled with beauty is music to the eye.

Always look at one's bright side before you listen with your eyes.

A slip of the hand
is not as slippery as
a slip of the tongue in the dark.

Sign softly and carry a big stick in your belt.

Show me your hand
and I will tell you
your school.

There are three sides
to every communication —
your side, my side
and the right side.

A new sign today is better than two empty hands tomorrow.

Rearm yourself now and then during an argument.

Signs speak louder than words.

Point only where
you can put your finger on it.

Hands-on experience is your best teacher.

A cracked floor can never pound true.

Many hands make light work of interpreting.

Signing and mudslinging do not mix.

The only difference between a fool's handiwork and a wise one's handwork is "i."

Double-signing is for politicians.

Anything signed more than a handful is wasted.

It goes without saying anyone can sign.

Handsome
is a beautiful signer.

A seesign is as good as a hearsay.

One eyewitness
is better than ten seesigns.

The ingredients of wisdom
are open eyes,
closed hands and silent mouth.

News when signed covers North, East, West and South.

Signs are
inner thoughts
coated with emotion
that quietly seep out.

Be original
or be second-hand.

Opportunity flashes but once.

The vibrating wheel gets the grease.

Do not bite the hand that signs to you.

Break the ice and
your hands will not get cold.

Eloquence smiles on those who sign with elegance.

Keep a poker face, and play your hands wisely.

Touch to hear the tone.

Uncover each new sign and ignorance will scurry away.

Give a Deafie space, and he will give you atmosphere.

Fores unheard beget foreheadaches.

The bigger the tree that falls,
the greater the pound.

Signing and silence rarely go hand-in-hand.

Find some street lights, and you will find some happy moths.

A signing Hearie flies like a firefly among moths.

Sleeves are there to keep one's signing discreet.

Redundancy
takes care of a broken finger.

Keep your fingernails filed, and your signs will come to the point quicker.

Your arms and mouth
are attached
to the front of your body
so you can watch what you say.

Wise is she
who has a handle
on her signing.

Hearie candor, discreetly put;
Deafie candor, bluntly put.

An innocent question answered unwittingly begets you an innocent answer.

Sign on or sign off.

Always put Deafies in good light.

Terps come in pairs,
for it takes two to tango.

Before you open your mouth, think aloud.

Forehanded is forearmed.

Captions
are as open as
they are closed.

Always put your drinks out of arm's way.

Signs are to eyes
what words are to ears.

An arc well taught will grow full circle.

A hearing-ear dog is a Deafie's best friend.

A deaf dog is still man's best friend.

Talking with two Hearies
at a right angle
makes a right triangle.

A Deafie is known by the company she keeps.

Old handshapes die hard.

Signing
brings on signing.

Wear your deafness as a peacock wears his colorful feathers.

Sign slowly, for the hand is quicker than the eye.

A moon
always shows its best side
when it casts
its full shadow behind.

Read between the fingers.

There are two sides
to every signed story —
the right one and
the left-handed.

Mainstreaming is no minor river.

Handwork
is signing the right thing
at the right time.

Out of signs,
out on two limbs.

Hindsight will tell you not to turn your back while talking.

When in the Deaf world,
do as the Deafies do.

Tap or dance around.

Different Deafies, different strokes.

A pause in one's signing
makes room
for a blink from another.

News flash is a phone call in the middle of the night.

Like the sea,
eyes always seek their own level.

Where there is a shadow,
there is a sunny side.

There is no love spell
sweeter than
signing sweet nothings
under the palm of
your lover's hand.

Without lids, tired ears;
With lids, fresh eyes.

Too many hands spoil the interpretation.

Fingernails
are put there to hammer
one's point home.

It pays to listen, but it costs nothing to see.

May your happy waves of signs splash over hard rocks of words.

One upplauding arm has the upper hand over clapping with one hand.

Sign up or ship out.

Tap one in a Deafie crowd and watch it multiply in waves.

Ears are noses
tucked inside the head
to sniff out sounds.

All signs
point to the big picture.

Wear a pair of deafing aids, and you will see.

The Deafie who laughs last, laughs best.

Unexpected Deafie encounters breed
unexpected Hearie reactions.

Sight makes right,
for seeing is believing.

As is the signer,
so is the signing.

Treat one and all alike – issue us the ticket or cop out.

Great signs
make a moving performance.

Shouting at a Deafie is like barking up the wrong tree.

A train of thought on fast lips is hard to catch.

Do not count your signs before they are used.

The sense
that has the lightest touch
goes the farthest.

Eyes are more prominent than ears.

Look out for punches in punchlines.

Face where
your walking feet face.

A good pair of eyes
will tire out
a hundred pairs of arms.

One is odd, two is even, three is one odd too many.

Look a Deafie in the eye,
and you will find a true soul.

A pound has a nice ring to it.

Even bad ears
hold up glasses for bad eyes.

One hand watches the other.

Signs spaced out come out well-paced.

Apologies
will not bring back the train.

Signs liberate words from the mouth.

A handscape
is a landscape fingerpainted.

Space well signed abhors a vacuum.

Perfect feedback, perfect speech.

Hand or mouth,
never judge a Deafie.

Air is rarer around great signers.

Absence makes
the deaf grow fonder.

A wide path is a happy one.

Hammer your signs
on the anvil of your imagination
until they spark.

Let what you cannot hear enhance what you can do.

A good expression
carries good face value.

Sign and sign alike.

Doubt frowns on those who smile their way out.

A picture signed is worth a thousand spoken words.

Look both ways –
even on a one-way street.

See no evil,
feel no evil,
sign no evil.

Two arms, two elbows,
two wrists, two hands,
two thumbs, eight fingers,
thirty joints —
what a moveable feast for the eye!

Signs your mirror mirrors, your memory memorizes.

The Hearie who closes his ears is a sound barrier.

A molehill signed is bigger than a mountain spoken.

The lip is the tip of an iceberg;
The rest is the body.

The one who watches is the one who understands.

Words when signed spring from one dimension to three.

Snooping has no place in TTY space.

Two wrong signs do not make a right sign.

There is no use
in talking to the back of
a Deafie's eyeballs.

The way to a Deafie's heart is through your hands.

Signs get to the point faster than words.

Never give Deafies the silent treatment.

Easier signed than done.

For a stronger accent,
roll up your sleeves.

Lipreading is
the fine art of navigating
a narrow mouth and
its stream of thoughts.

All eyes
make great listeners.

Hear today, gone tomorrow.

You cannot wash spots off a Deafie Dalmatian.

Signs without polish bounce off glazed eyes.

One world fades away and
another opens up
for the Late-Deafened.

Learn to sign,
lest your thoughts are
lost on lips.

The Deafie world is a stage — turn on all the lights!

Sign like honey,
and others will find you
finger-lickin' good.

Fences are never too high for the hard-of-hearing to jump off.

Put down Deafies' arms,
and they will be up in arms.

Cued speech is signing in the cheek.

Bored ears or eyes,
in one and out the other.

You can lead a Deafie
to a hearing-aid,
but you cannot make him hear.

Strike
while your sign is hot.

Two hands
are better than
one tongue.

Sign by sign
you are home.

Deafies in glass houses have the best view and no privacy.

Anything worth signing is worth signing well.

A caged Deafie longs for the clubs.

Fluency is but sign deep.

Every Deafie mother's child is hand-some.

Signs in print are signs caught frozen in time.

You may talk,
but keep your hands busy.

A proper sign in time saves nine.

Like Deafie parents, like Deafie children.

Where there are Deafies there will be signs.

Silent majority of yesteryear is silent no more.

Relay operators give
your fingers voice
and your eyes ears.

Signing and talking make strange bedfellows.

Take nothing at face value;
Step back and
see the big picture.

Everything that can be seen, can be done.

Culture your Deaf culture,
or it dilutes.

May the sun of happiness never set on your Deafie world.

Index of Proverbial Keywords

A

Abhors 181
Abilities 9
Absence 185
Accent 209
Air 184
Alarm 28
Alike 162
All eyes 211
All signs 156
Aloud 118
Angle 126
Answer 114
Anvil 187
Anyone 86
Apologies 178
Applause 22
Arc 123
Arguing 59
Argument 76
Arm 152
Arm's way 121
Arms 111, 171, 220
Atmosphere 102
Attached 111
Attracts 42

B

Bad ears 175
Barking 164
Barrier 197
Beautiful 87
Beauty 69
Bedfellows 239
Believing 160
Belt 72
Best 132, 227
Best friend . . .124, 125
Big eyes 14
Big picture . . .156, 240
Bird 12
Bite (vb.) 96
Blinds (vb.) 19
Blink 142
Bluntly put 113
Book 44
Bored 222
Borrowing 7
Brain 6
Break (vb.) 97
Bright side 35, 70
Brings on 129
Broken finger 109
Busy 233

C

Caged 229
Candor 113
Capabilities 9
Capabled 21
Captions 120
Cheap 17
Cheek 221
Child 3, 231
Children 24, 235
Clapping 152
Clear (vb.) 28
Clip (vb.) 32
Closed 90, 120
Clubs 229
Cold 97
Colors 25
Communication 74
Company 127
Cop out 162
Costs nothing 150
Count (vb.) 166
Cracked floor 80
Crowd 154
Cued speech 221
Culture 242

D

Dalmatian 213
Dance 140
Dark 71
Deaf (adj.) 5, 10, 16, 31
. . . 125, 139, 159, 242
Deaf (n.) 40, 185
Deaf culture 242
Deaf dog 125
Deaf ears 5
Deaf world 139
Deaf-impaired 60
Deafing aids 157

Deafness 52, 130
Deep 230
Designer 15, 27
Die hard 128
Difference 83
Different 141
Dilutes 242
Dimension 201
Disabled 21
Disarm 27
Discovers 2
Discreet 108
Discreetly put 113
Do 139, 188
Dog 124, 125
Done 208, 241
Door knob 10
Double-signing 84
Doubt 191
Drinks 121

E

Ears . . .5, 122, 147, 155
  168, 175, 197, 222, 238
Easier signed 208
Easy to see 45
Eat 48
Eloquence 98
Emotion 92
Empty 75
Empty-handedness . .13
Encounters 159
Enhance 188

Even 172
Everything 241
Evil 194
Experience 79
Expression 189
Eye 131, 173, 195
Eyeballs 204
Eyes . . .7, 14, 16, 47, 55
  . . . . .70, 90, 122, 144
  . . .147, 168, 171, 175
  . . .211, 214, 222, 238
Eyewitness 89

F

Face (vb.) 11, 170
Face value 189, 240
Fades away 215
Fall (vb.) 5
Falls 104
Farthest 167
Fast lips 165
Faster 54, 206
Feast 195
Feathers 130
Feedback 182
Feet 170
Fences 219
Filed 110
Fine art 210
Finer gift 3
Finger 78, 109
Finger-lickin' 218
Fingernails . . . 110, 149
Fingerpainted 180

Fingers 49, 133
  . . . . 195, 238
Firefly 107
Flash 143
Flashes 94
Flies 107
Floor 28, 80
Flowers 63
Fluency 230
Fly 24, 32
Fonder 185
Fool 83
Forearmed 119
Fores 103
Forgotten 58
Fresh 147
Friend 34, 124, 125
Front 111
Frowns (vb.) 191
Frozen 232
Full 39
Full circle 123
Full shadow 132

G

Gear 6
Gift 3
Glass houses 227
Glasses 175
Glazed eyes 214
Glib terps 57
Golden 30
Golfers 61
Gone 212

Good 88, 218
Good expression . . .189
Good light 116
Good pair 171
Good sign 68
Gossip 66
Grease 95
Great 163, 184, 211
Greater 18, 49, 104
Grow 123
Grow fonder 185
Guessture 58

H

Half-empty 21
Hammer 149, 187
Hand 20, 44, 71, 73
. . . . .96, 131, 146
. . . . . . .152, 176 183
Hand-in-hand 105
Hand-me-down 3
Hand-some 231
Handful 85
Handicap 61
Handiwork 83
Handle 112
Hands . .6, 39, 47, 52, 6
. . . . .75, 81, 90, 97, 99
148, 195, 205, 225, 233
Hands full 39
Hands still 67
Hands-on 79

Handscape 180
Handshapes 128
Handsome 87
Handwork 83, 136
Happiness 243
Happy medium 58
Happy moths 106
Happy one 23, 186
Happy waves 151
Hard knocks 23
Hard rocks 151
Hard to catch 165
Hard-of-hearing . . .219
Harder 59
Head 67, 155
Hear 100, 188, 212, 223
Hearie (adj.)24, 113, 159
Hearie (n.) 43, 60
. . . . .107, 197
Hearies 126
Hearing-aid 223
Hearing-ear dog . . .124
Hearing-impaired . . .60
Hearly bird 12
Hearsay 88
Heart 205
High 219
Hindsight 138
Home 149, 226
Honey 218
Hot 224
Houses 227
Hundred 171

I

"i" 83
Ice 97
Iceberg 199
Ignorance 101
Illuminates 19
Imagination 187
In gear 6
In one 222
In pairs 117
In print 232
In time 232, 234
Ingredients 90
Inner thoughts 92
Innocent 114
Interest 7
Interpretation 148
Interpreting 81
Invisible 52

J

Joints 195
Judge (vb.) 183
Jump off 219

K

Keep 108, 233
Keeps 33, 65, 127
Knob 10
Knocks (n.) 23
Known 127

L

Landscape 180
Late-Deafened 215
Laughs 158
Lead (vb.) 40, 223
Learn 216
Learned 68
Left-handed 134
Level 144
Liberate 179
Lids 147
Light . . 25, 51, 54, 116
Light work 81
Lightest touch 167
Lights 66, 106, 217
Limbs 137
Lip 199
Lip service 57
Lipreading 210
Lips 38, 165, 216
Listen 70, 150
Listeners 211
Listens 16
Little 26
Look (n.) 4
Look (vb.) 193
Look at 70
Loose lips 38
Louder 77
Love 31
Love spell 146

M

Mainstreaming 135
Majority 237
Many eyes 47
Many hands . . . 81, 148
Marry 43
Medium 58
Memory 196
Mightier 46
Minor 135
Mirror 196
Molehill 198
Money 20, 64, 65
Moon 132
Mother's child 231
Moths 106, 107
Motion 6
Mountain 198
Mouth 49, 90, 118
. . . . 179, 183, 210
Moveable 195
Moving 163
Mudslinging 82
Multiply 154
Music 11, 69

N

Navigating 210
News 91, 143
Night 143
Nine 234
Noise 30
Noses 155
Nothing 240

O

Odd 172
One hand 152
One-way 193
Open (adj.) 90, 120
Open (vb.) 52, 118
Opens up 215
Operators 238
Opportunity 94
Original 93
Out of signs 137
Out the other 222

P

Pair 157, 171
Pairs 117, 171
Palm 146
Parents 235
Path 186
Pause 142
Pays 150
Peacock 130
Perfect 182
Performance 163
Phone call 143
Picture 156, 240
Picture signed 192
Place 62, 202
Point (n.) . 110, 149, 206
Point (vb. 78, 156

Poker face 99
Polish 214
Politicians 84
Potatoes 14
Pound (n.) . . .104, 174
Pound (vb.) 41, 80
Pound the floor 28
Print 232
Privacy 227
Prominent 168
Proper sign 234
Punches 169
Pure silence 37
Put down 220

Q

Question 114
Quicker 110, 131
Quietly 92

R

Rainbow colors 25
Rarer 184
Reach out 34
Reactions 159
Read (vb.) 133
Rearm 76
Recharges 37
Redundancy 109
Relay operators . . . 238
Repels 42

Resign 50
Right 160, 203
Right angle 126
Right side 35, 74
Right thing 136
Ring 174
River 135
Road 36
Rocks 151
Room 142

S

Sans signs 15
School 23, 73
Scurry 101
Sea 144
Second-hand 93
Seeing 160
Seep (vb.) 92
Seesign 88
Seesigns 89
Sense 18, 167
Shadow 145
Ship out 153
Shoulder tap 4
Shouting 164
Show me 73
Shut 47
Side 74, 132, 145
Side-by-side 40
Sides 134
Sight 160

Sign alike 190
Sign deep 230
Sign on 115
Sign slowly 131
Sign softly 72
Sign up 153
Signed 8, 198, 201
Signed story 134
Signer 15, 87, 161
Signing (adj.) 107
Signing (n.) . .129, 239
Signing (vb.) 136
Silence . . .30, 37, 105
Silence sprinkled . . .69
Silent 65, 90, 237
Silent treatment . . .207
Silvery 30
Sink (vb.) 38
Sleeping 37
Sleeves 108, 209
Slip 71
Slowly 131
Small part 10
Smile 4, 191
Smiles (vb.) 98
Sniff out 155
Snooping 202
Snore 43
Soft and sweet 48
Soul 173
Sound barrier 197
Sound sleep 53

Soundless 53	Talking . . .138, 204 239	Travels faster 54
Space 102, 181	Talks 64	Treat (vb.) 162
Spaced out 177	Tango 117	Treatment 207
Spark 187	Tap (n.) 4	Tree 104, 164
Speech 182	Tap (vb.) 140, 154	Triangle 126
Splash over 151	Taught 123	True 80, 173
Spoil 148	Teach 3, 64	TTY 202
Spoken 198	Teacher 33, 79	Turn out 66
Spoken words 192	Tell 73, 138	Turn your back 138
Spots 213	Ten 49, 89	Twice 62
Stage 217	Terps 57, 117	Two 75, 117, 172
Stand under 51	Thought 165	Two arms 195
Stars unheard 45	Thoughts . .92, 210, 216	Two hands 225
Steep 17	Thousand 192	Two Hearies 126
Stick 72	Three . .74, 172, 201	Two sides 134
Strange 239	Ticket 162	
Stream 210	Time .68, 136, 232, 234	**U**
Street 56, 193	Tip 199	
Street lights 106	Tiptoe 43	Uncover 101
Strike (vb.) 224	Tire out 171	Understand 51
Strikes twice 62	Tired ears 147	Understands 200
Strokes 141	Today 75, 212	Unexpected 159
Stronger 209	Tomorrow 75, 212	Unheard 45, 103
Sum 49	Tone 100	Unsigned 8
Sun 243	Tongue 71, 225	Unwittingly 114
Sunny 145	Too high 219	Up in arms 220
Sweet nothings 146	Too many 47, 172	Upper hand 152
	Topsoil 63	Upplauding 152
T	Total 49	Upplause 22
Tabletops 63	Touch 34, 100, 167	
Talk (n.) 17, 56	Train 165, 178	**V**
Talk (vb.) 39, 233	Traveled 36	Vacuum 181
		Value 189, 240

Vibrating 95	Wisdom 90	Your belt 72
View 227	Wise (adj.) .67, 83, 112	Your body 111
Voice 238	Wise (n.) 29	Your brain 6
	Wisely 99	Your child 3
W	With elegance 98	Your deafness 130
Walk (vb.) 40	Without lids 147	Your drinks 121
Walking feet 170	Without polish ...214	Your eyes 70, 238
Wash (vb.) 213	Without saying 86	Your finger 78
Wasted 85	Word 12, 46	Your fingernails ...110
Watch 26, 111, 154	Words 77, 122, 151	Your fingers 238
Watches 176, 200	....179, 192, 201, 206	Your hand 20, 73
Waves 151, 154	Work 81	Your hands ..6, 47, 52
Way 121, 191, 205	World 2, 65, 139	........99, 205, 233
Ways 193	........215, 217, 243	Your imagination ..187
Wear 130, 157	Worlds 24	Your memory 196
Well signed 181	Worth signing 228	Your mirror 196
Well taught 123	Worth two 44	Your money 20
Well-paced 177	Wrists 195	Your mouth 118
Wheel 95	Wrong signs 203	Your side 74
White light 25	Wrong tree 164	Your sign 224
Whole thing 10		Your signs 48, 110
Wide path 186	**Y**	...........166, 187
Window 19	Yesteryear 237	Your sleeves 209
Windows 55	Your back 138	Your thoughts 216
Wings 24, 32		Yourself 76

About the Author

KEN GLICKMAN is a widely recognized figure in the American Deaf community and known for his humorous contributions to Deaf culture. His journey to becoming the guru of DEAFology unfolded during his 11 years as a profoundly deaf student at Clarke School for the Deaf in his native state of Massachusetts. He then moved on to graduate from Dartmouth College *magna cum laude* with High Distinction in Psychology. This somehow prepared him to join IBM in 1977 as a computer programmer. He taught programming and computer graphics at National Technical Institute for the Deaf (NTID) at RIT (1980-81) and at Gallaudet University (1985-86) under IBM's Faculty Loan Program.

In 1987, Glickman left IBM to establish *DEAFinitely Yours Studio* and has been griping about the tax forms ever since. He has published two books, *DEAFinitions* (1986) and *More DEAFinitions!* (1989), and is completing work on a third volume, *DEAFinitions Galore!*

Ken frequently takes his comedy show on the road in the form of two crash courses on Deaf culture, DEAFology 101 and 201. In these, Ken as "Prof Glick" supplies his own unique brand of quirky logic and keen observation, drawn from his life experience not just as a deaf individual, but also as an author, a desktop publisher, a webmaster, a poet, a magician, a wordsmith and a comedian. In 1999, he was seized with an extremely rare, compulsive condition that compelled him to jot down every passing thought and insight about deaf culture into proverb form. This book is the result. He may be cured now, although you'll have to try one of his DEAFology courses to determine this for yourself.

He lives in Silver Spring, Maryland, with Debbie and their loyal dog, Star.

Deaf Proverbs — A Proverbial Professor's Points to Ponder

Ideal for Deaf Studies
Perfect for Gifts
Great for Your Coffee Table!

This book is available in both softcover and hardcover. Priced at $14.95 and $19.95, respectively, they can be purchased from ***DEAFinitely Yours Studio*** (add $4.00 for shipping/handling) or from Ken's website at http://www.deafology.com.

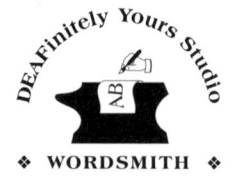

❖ WORDSMITH ❖

DEAFinitely Yours Studio

9201 Long Branch Parkway
Silver Spring, Maryland 20901-3642 USA
301-434-4040 TTY 301-434-6626 FAX
800-735-2258 Maryland Relay Service
E-Mail: ProfGlick@deafology.com
Website: http://www.deafology.com